MEN,
HOW MUCH DO
YOU REALLY
LOVE YOUR
FAMILY?

DURAND C. SPRUILL

Published in New York by Yarrah Properties, Inc.

Printed in the United States of America

ISBN 978-0-578-14660-7

(1) Men—Health
(2) Men—Family
(3) Fatherhood—Religion

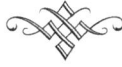

*This book is dedicated to the memory of
my loving father, Harry J. Spruill and my
brilliant older brother, Ameil H. Spruill.*

MANY PEOPLE CONTRIBUTED TO THIS BOOK & I LOVE ALL OF YOU.
THERE ARE A FEW I WOULD LIKE TO PUBLICLY THANK:

*To my rock, my support system and the love of
my life for the past 25 years, my wife. You refused to let me
'zone out' into depression. Baby, I love you with all of my heart.*

*To my other support, my mother.
You have weathered many storms yet still you
stand strong in your faith and love. Love you mom.*

*To my editors Crystal Joseph and Dr. Talonda Thomas,
thank you very much for your time and support.
Dr. Thomas, I so appreciate your consistent encouragement.
Crystal, you are exceptionally talented, I am glad to have you as
my friend. And to my book designer Naomi Caesar, you have
a gift and I thank you for sharing it with me.*

*I would like to give a special thanks to Beatrice Page and
Reilly Elizabeth Bashir for being photographed on the cover.*

I also would like to thank the photographer, Anthony Mitchell.

ABOUT THE AUTHOR

Durand has worked in the healthcare industry for over fifteen years as a Physical Rehabilitation Evaluator. He received his collegiate education in business at Howard University in Washington, D.C.

Durand is writing this book based on his experience with prostate cancer. He is not a physician nor is he an expert in the field. He simply hopes to encourage others, by telling His story, to get examined early.

Durand is married and has two children. He and his wife have been members of Bethel Gospel Tabernacle Incorporated, where Bishop Roderick Caesar is the Senior Pastor, for over twenty-two years. Durand has been serving as an ordained deacon for eight years.

CONTENTS

INTRODUCTION

Men, one of the ways we love our family is by taking care of ourselves and getting regular checkups. The stakes are too high for us to say that we're too busy or that we feel fine and do not need a physical. We have too much to lose if we take this gamble.

In regards to an ailment that could have been treated, would you rather end up as a cold lifeless corpse or a warm-blooded, living being?

The choice is yours to make and was mine.

DISBELIEF

My report from biopsy was printed today. I have cancer in my prostate. My feeling is one of shock and disbelief.

Hi, my name is Durand C. Spruill and this is my story. Please allow me to indulge with my personal history before I address the title of this book. I married my lovely wife when I was 26 years old and we have been happily married for 20 years.

I work out three times a week. I took red meat out of my diet the day after I got married. I just lost the taste for it. As a birthday gift to myself, I get annual physicals. This year when I go, my PSA is relatively high. A PSA is a blood sample test which indicates the condition of your prostate, according to medical practitioners. In other words, it is a screen for prostate cancer. This year my PSA has flared up to four. Normally, it should be around two for someone my age. I was in my forties. My doctor refers me to an urologist who conducts a digital exam and finds that everything is normal. A couple of months later, I take another PSA exam and my number is back down to two. I am feeling great. I am 5'10", 185 pounds and I am not on any medication. I go on my merry way.

Next year in the spring, I went for my yearly physical and my PSA is up to 5, which is slightly above normal for someone my age. No problem, I say to myself. It could be something I ate. I will come back in a couple of months and get re-tested. Well, this time when I get re-tested, the PSA number remained the same. My primary care doctor referred me to an urologist who I strongly disliked. He made absolutely no eye contact with me nor did he explain anything to me. I felt as though all of the men in the waiting room were nothing but cattle being paraded through his little farm. There was no connection so I chose a different urologist next time, one with whom I was more comfortable (he also had smaller fingers). My new urologist Dr. M., suggested I get a biopsy based on my family history. Are you kidding me? I have never had a medical procedure in my life. I am as healthy as a horse! I have no medical symptoms, but to put everyone's concerns to rest including my own, I decide to go through with the biopsy.

I lost a close buddy to prostate cancer a couple months ago. He died at age 52. By the time he went for his examinations and treatments, he was too far gone. I also lost my Dad to prostate cancer at age 63. On his death bed, my father said that he knew he had a medical problem years ago but did not do any intervention. At the urging of my wife, and the thoughts of the two previously mentioned losses, I was motivated to have my biopsy procedure. I did not know what to expect. A year ago when I was about to be digitally examined by my first urologist, I questioned his practice of medicine and suggested he was behind the technology times. Certainly in this day and age an X-Ray or CAT scan should be sufficient to detect cancer of the prostate. I did not understand why he had to feel my prostate with his finger through my rectum. I found out later that this is done to

check the normalcy of the prostate size. This is
an emotional problem because men do not share
and communicate what to expect from your first
prostate exam. It was a culture shock to me to
be examined digitally. Afterwards, I went home
and sat in my living room alone in disbelief. I
do believe I was traumatized because all my life
I was taught the anus had one function, and that
was to be used as an exit – not for anything else,
including a medical examination cavity. I have
been told generally speaking, when a woman sees
a gynecologist for the first time, she is prepared
by other women as to what to expect. With men,
there is no preparation from other men. You are
treading in unknown territory. It is on you to figure
it out. One of the strategies is to use a relaxing
breathing technique similar to that which is used
in Lamaze classes. That technique consists of
breathing in through your nose and out through
your mouth. This will hopefully help relax you.
Another strategy is meditation to the point you
are so relaxed and do not feel physically present.
For example: although you are in a doctor's
office, think yourself into a peaceful place. I like

to picture myself on a Caribbean beach. Others like to pray. Some focus on scriptures. The choice is yours. It is not my intention to scare you but to have honest dialogue with you.

RESULTS OF THE PROCEDURE

Today is the morning of the prostate biopsy. A plastic camera with one needle is inserted into my rectum in order to reach my prostate. Blood is drawn from twelve different sections of my prostate. Though the whole process took one minute, it honestly felt like fifteen. I didn't actually feel pain, but I felt the pinch of each needle pricks.

As I left the doctor's office, I had to walk very slowly. I gingerly entered the car and turned it on. Driving was okay until I hit that first bump. The pain went through my entire core. Actually, it went from my rectum to the pit of my stomach. After that, I realized that I had to rise up in my car seat in order to avoid all of the other bumps on my way home.

The mental trauma continued when I got home. I sat and once again tried to process what I had just went through. Thank God for my wife.

She helped make it much easier.

After awhile, I went to the bathroom and was shocked. Blood was in my stool. It looked like red clay in the toilet. There were a couple of blood clots in my urine and I felt sore for the rest of the day.

My son was thirteen years old. I had to be strong and brave for him. I teach my son to only fear God and bad decisions that can end up with negative results. Going to the doctor and taking care of myself physically was my way of showing him that not doing those things can end up with negative results. I informed him that real courageous men get their prostates examined. The easy thing to do is not to have the exam or biopsy done. I should say it's easy to make that decision on the front end, but may be disastrous on the 'back end' (no pun intended). It takes courage to face the unknown as well as being uncomfortable, but I did it for my family because I love them and I want to be there for them. Indirectly, I did it for myself, but I was never the main focus. At least, that's how I felt.

I kept thinking of my deceased friend's advice

to a group of men while on the bus of a fishing trip. He urged us to have a prostate exam. That, along with my father's premature death heavily influenced my decision to get the procedure done.

The result of my biopsy came back positive for cancer. I said to Dr. M., there has to be some mistake. I don't eat red meat and I do aerobics three times a week. The doctor responded there are three variables to look at in determining the origin of cancer. The following are in no particular order. The first is diet – the kinds of food you eat. Green leafy vegetables are better for your health than fatty, acidic foods (raw spinach instead of a steak). Second is your environment - minimize your stress by exercising. The third is your genetic makeup – what chemistry you have inherited (my father had prostate cancer so it is in my family). Unfortunately, your genetic makeup has nothing to do with age. It is the cards in life you have been dealt. Dr. M. informed me that a thirty-five year old man was diagnosed with the same illness the same time I received my diagnosis. What blows my mind is the fact that I had no symptoms whatsoever. As I stated in the beginning, Dr. M. said I should be thankful I have women (my mom and wife) in my life who push me to get checkups.

Moving on, now I have to go through a series of bone scans and cat scans to see if the cancer has spread and also determine the stage. I am singing to myself 'praises to God' as I go through my scans. The challenging part is waiting six days for the results. It was the most solemn six days of my life and played on my emotions. I did not know the results concerning the stage. I did not know if I would live to see my daughter graduate from college or live long enough to see my son grow up into manhood. I prayed seriously, earnestly for divine healing. My results came back Stage 1 out of four stages. Let me explain: Stage 1 & 2 – Curable // Stage 3 & 4 - Controllable but filled with pain and suffering such as bone pain, paralysis, etc. (Please note: I am a Christian so I definitely believe that miracles do happen at any stage). The CAT scan revealed that the cancer was contained in the prostate and had not spread. I didn't receive this information until after Thanksgiving which put a dark cloud over that holiday but we definitely had a Merry Christmas. Hallelujah!

Dr. M. said the choice of treatments was mine to make whether I should go for the surgery (Radical Prostatectomy) or radiation. The difference is clear: one involves surgery and the subsequent removal of the prostate. The other involves radiation with a possibility of the cancer returning. I could also choose to do nothing, as my father did, and run the risk of the cancer spreading to my bones.

THY WILL BE DONE

After being diagnosed, I had a "Gethsemane" experience. Father, please let this cup pass from me. Nevertheless, not my will but ... Oh who am I kidding? I really did want MY will to be done. I didn't want this cancer. I did not want to go through this situation. Eventually, I came to myself and began praising God and said "nevertheless, THY will be done".

I finally chose surgery and thank God for my friends. Monique offered to drive my wife to the hospital to visit me. Dee, who worked at the hospital, said she would make sure I would be well taken care of during my stay there. It took about a month before I made my decision to have the surgery. It is not for me to tell you what form of treatment to choose, whether it is holistic, surgery, or radiation. It is a personal choice. But I am strongly advocating that you get examined. Prostate cancer with early detection is treatable. Are there possible side effects with all of the different treatments? Sure. I just figured it was better for me to be around with possible side effects than not be around at all!

YOUR PRESENCE IS NEEDED

I knew I was needed to guide my son through manhood. I knew I was needed to teach my daughter how men think and operate. I knew I was needed to support my wife. I knew I was needed to provide wisdom and advice to my family. I knew I was needed, period. I made my decision based on my love for my family and I encourage you to do the same.

How do you feel about your family? Do you truly love them and want what is best for them? Have you ever had the chance and opportunity to hug your children and tell them that you love them? Have you been fortunate enough to love your spouse and express love to her? Well, I have. It does wonders for them. For the most part, the world is a cold, dark, and negative place. To come home to someone and have them hear, validate, and make you feel like you matter is a precious thing. The feeling is a double benefit because it is good to give out love to your family and to receive it. It adds to your character and gives you purpose. You become the anchor and driving force of all the goals that come out of your house. Your children and wife will be comfortable in coming to you with all their problems because they know that you genuinely love them and have shown it. It is good for you to be wanted and needed. Hence, I thought it would be a good idea for me to stick around.

Is it worth being a judge and rendering decisions and options of every case in your house? I would say yes. There is never a dull moment. When things get too hectic or overwhelming you have an advisor to lean upon and consult – your spouse. If you don't have a spouse, bounce things off your confidant.

Every sane person I know does not want to be sick. Today you can feel like Hercules. Tomorrow you may get a bad report from the doctor. Your love for yourself and for your family should determine or impact your response to the medical dilemma. If it is God's will for your time to die, then it is His will. However, if God has given you a second chance to live, as He has for me, then you should more than take care of the body He has given you by getting medical examinations. Also, if you are the appropriate age to have your prostate examined, by all means do it. If you're African-American, that age is 40. All others the age is 50. Early detection is curable and your family will love you for it. I encourage you to do it. How much do you honor your family's love?

BEFORE THE SURGERY

MONDAY: THREE DAYS BEFORE SURGERY

A coworker confesses to me just how blessed I am. She said I am blessed because I have legions of angels and Godly people to support and stand with me.

I'm medically cleared by the hospital and my primary physician. I'm on a liquid diet for four days.

WEDNESDAY: THE DAY BEFORE SURGERY

My sister and her husband pray for me over the telephone. My friend Kevin prays for me as well.

THURSDAY: THE DAY OF THE SURGERY

I had to be at the hospital by 9:30am. My mom came with me. I needed my wife to stay home so she could be there for my son.

The operation is scheduled at 1:00pm.

However, it did not occur until 4:30pm due to a backlog. I kissed my mom and sent her home to avoid the snowstorm that is about to begin. The operation took two and a half hours. I awaken after surgery feeling very sore and have a Foley catheter (urine bag) which I have to wear for three weeks. I am groggy and want to urinate but it feels as though I can't.

FRIDAY: DAY ONE AFTER SURGERY

There is a snow storm outside today. We got two and one-half FEET OF SNOW! Schools are closed because of this massive snow storm.

I call my family and tell them that I would see them tomorrow at discharge. I am groggy, in pain, and nauseous due to the medication. I am very weak, too weak to clean myself. Dee, my friend at the hospital, has to bathe me. I am moved by her compassion but also very humbled.

I got out of the bed on my own and walked around the hospital floor. I had to walk so that fluid wouldn't accumulate in my lungs resulting in pneumonia.

SATURDAY: DAY TWO AFTER SURGERY

My wife, mother, and brother pick me up this morning. There is still about two feet of snow on the ground. I have metal staples in my lower abdomen and each bump that we hit on the ride home is very agonizing.

TUESDAY: DAY FIVE AFTER SURGERY

I have been constipated since the surgery on Thursday. This morning I finally go to the bathroom. It is difficult and very painful. I am concerned because I don't want to pop the staples in my stomach.

There is an emotional and psychological aspect to facing the consequences of medical treatment. As an illustration, some women have large vaginas and some have small vaginas. Some women have small breasts and some have large breasts. Is a woman who has a small vagina and small breasts size any less than a woman with larger breasts and vagina? We know this could not be anything further from the truth. You have to know who you are. If you were born a woman, you are a woman. If you are born a man, you are a man - regardless of whether or not your reproductive organs are working properly or not. Thus, my manhood is not defined by the size of my penile organ or how well it is working. The reason why I am bringing this up is because one of the possible side effects, whether you get surgery or radiation, is erectile dysfunction (ED). I just figured it would be better for me to be around and give my children and possible grandchildren advice and guidance than placing emphasis on the possibility (it's not a definite side effect) of erectile dysfunction from the operation.

There is no medical surgery used to save your life that can or will change your birth identity. If a woman has one breast or both breasts removed, it does not negate her from being a woman. If a man has one testicle or both testicles removed, or becomes impotent, it does not negate him from being a man. A medical change in your life should not cause anyone to change from the person they were born to be.

Surgeries such as Radical Prostatectomy (removal of the prostate), Mastectomy (removal of a breast), as well as side effects such as impotence, do not define who you are. You may choose to have an organ removed for medical necessity. You may or may not have side effects from surgery or from radiation treatment. Either way, your body will need time to heal and adjust. You have to ask yourself, who are you doing it for?

THINGS TO EXPECT
WHILE IN THE HOSPITAL

When you are sick, you are so vulnerable physically, emotionally, and mentally. In the hospital, I did not think the same, feel the same or physically present the same person as I did when I was healthy. I wanted my independence and not being able to get it was very embarrassing.

Hospital employees, although overworked and understaffed, should be sensitive to this but sadly, this may not be true in some cases. The opposite is also true. There are some very mean patients admitted to the hospital. I feel compassion for the employees that must work with these mean people however they should remember that even this experience is very humbling for the vulgar patients as well.

Once I was discharged from the hospital, I was out on disability for 3 months convalescing at home.

THE BENCHMARK

Today is my three year anniversary. I lost about ten pounds when I was home convalescing. It took about six months before I was able to do a regimen of 20 sit ups and pushups. Now three years past my surgery, I've resumed my normal regimen of 100 sit ups and 50 pushups. My urologist tells me after three years, I am out of the woods.

During the first year my lower abdomen was tender and my sense of balance was off. During the second year I started feeling more like my old self and my natural weight returned. After three years, my overall health is good. I am ten pounds over my desired weight. I have a healthy appetite and I am not on any prescription medications. I move a bit slower now than I did three years ago. I do not know if it is due to the cancer operation or the fact that I am getting older. What I can tell you is each year I am feeling better and performing extracurricular activities better. The main thing is that I am here and alive with control of my faculties. Do I wish I never drank from this cup? Probably. However, I believe I was chosen and although I don't know why, I can testify that God is a healer. Because of Him, I was able to handle this ordeal and so can you. We all have crosses to bear in life, and this was mine. I also believe I was chosen to help other men realize that a physical sickness or challenge does not define or diminish your manhood. How do I know? My manhood is demonstrated and proven every day when I engage with my family. If you asked me if I made the right decision to do something about my health, my answer would be absolutely!

Today I met with my urologist after three years post-surgery. For the past three years I had to see him every quarter to check and see if the cancer cells were growing back. Today the report is good. Now, I only have to see the doctor twice a year. The doctor states three, five, and ten years are benchmarks. As each year passes, it is less likely that the cancer will return. I read somewhere that cancer exists in an acidic environment — that is toxic overload, emotional stress and an acidic forming diet such as sugar, white flour, coffee, soda, etc. I drink a green drink (blended barley plants and wheat grass) every day and try to keep my diet as alkaline as possible – that is filled with mostly fruits, seeds, lentils and green vegetables. In the past three years as I have gone for my doctor examinations, the men that I see in the waiting room look much older than me. I am concerned that not enough younger men are going for prostate examinations. Remember age 40 is the minimum age for African-Americans.

I wished we lived in a world where there was no pain or sickness but unfortunately, that is not the case. Prostate cancer does not have to be a death sentence if detected early and detection is obtained through examination. Your life and the contributions to your family matter more than the possible side effects of cancer treatment. Modern day medicine has different options which can address the possible side effects.

MY REASONS
FOR EXAMINATION

My children don't expect to be belittled
when they walk through the doors of our house.
My children don't expected to be hit, kicked, or
cussed out when they walk through the doors
of our house. My children don't expect to be
ignored or overlooked when they are home.
And I suspect your children don't expect that
either. On the contrary, our children expect to be
loved and engaged when they are home. They
want physical interaction and verbal exchange
and attention when they are home. At the risk
of sounding traditional, after their mother has
worked a full shift, whether in or outside of the
home and prepares dinner, the least I could do is
be Mr. Coach, Mr. Entertainment, Mr. Confidant,
Mr. Friend and most importantly Dad.

I don't expect my household to be perfect. I
expect there to be turmoil at times. I don't expect

that the wife, the kids, and I will always agree. However, I don't expect my home environment to be vastly different than how people treat each other on the streets. It has been said the world is a dog eat dog world. I want my home to be supportive. Don't you want the same? When things are off kilter I will set the tone and get it all back into balance. All of the above helped influenced my decision to have surgery.

I did not want my children to become negative statistics. I wanted to be around to encourage them to excel. I wanted them to have a positive influence on other kids they knew and encountered. I wanted my children to represent all the good that is inside me and strive to be better. I still had so much to teach them. I wanted my legacy to be carried on through them. I wanted them to be able to stand on their own two feet, to be able to support themselves and earn a living. I felt my mission was not complete and I had more to offer. I believe every man who considers himself a real man and a real father, wants what is best for his children. But if that man is not around to teach, provide wisdom and influence, who do we leave the responsibility too?

My daughter was in college studying abroad in China. I chose not to tell her about my ordeal because I did not want to interfere with her studies. She was focusing on her studies. I wanted to live to show her what to look for in a man and not settle or lower her standards.

I wanted to live to teach my son about manhood because this is my job as a father. I wanted to show him how to treat a woman and how to choose a wife. I wanted to show my son how to deal with temptation and the consequences of yielding to it. I wanted to show him how to make decisions. I wanted to be around to pour into his life. I wanted to be alive to set boundaries for my son, otherwise he might not respect boundaries in the future which could cost him his life or freedom. I would not be around or I did not want to take the chance of not being around if I had not taken care of my prostate problem.

We all have specific challenges in life. I believe each person is given that challenge based on his or her level of tolerance to handle the situation. I believe we go through things so that

God can use us to be a blessing to others. You might ask "how in the world could my illness be a blessing to others?" The first way is by the mere fact that I am willing to discuss a private personal topic and be honest about myself within this book. Hopefully, this discussion will encourage men to get their prostate examined. Hopefully, men will realize there is no stigma attached and that they can go on with their lives. Second, I want men to know that there is no reason to be fearful about getting their prostate examined.

Since I am being truthful, I must tell you that I prayed to God concerning my medical situation. I did not rely solely on my own strength but I looked through the eyes of faith and knew that God was working it out on my behalf for his glory. It was not about me or my situation, but it was and still is about my Heavenly Father receiving all of the adoration and praise that I can give.

When I was diagnosed with cancer, I knew this was a defining moment in my life. Not so much that I had a cancerous prostate – people get sick every day – but it was my response to this ordeal that made it a defining moment. I could ignore the situation and wish it would go away (wishing is only good in fairy tales) or I could make some lifestyle changes.

MY DAD & I

My relationship with my dad was excellent. I loved and respected him so very much. He was my hero. He was the quintessential definition of what a man should be. My dad was tall, athletic, and handsome. My dad possessed the wisdom of Solomon and the swagger of John Shaft (an African-American superhero – if you are not familiar with 'Shaft' then imagine someone you may know with a silky smoothness and you will know the style of my father). But what stood out mostly about my father was his character. He was a man of integrity. His word was his bond. He could be trusted and he lived a righteous life. He did not try to be like anyone else. He was comfortable with himself. He knew who he was and who he belonged to! He did not squander his earnings. He made sure we had food on the table and clothes on our backs. He worked two jobs. He paid for my college education and my siblings too. I knew how to trust and depend on God because of the kind of man my father was. He was my first Sunday school teacher. His life had purpose. As I put pen to paper, tears are welling up in my eyes because I know how blessed I was to have him in my life. When my dad passed, I did not inherit a mansion or a lot of money, however he did leave my mother with a fully paid home (no mortgage) and debt free. But I inherited something much more valuable - a rich legacy. The only regrettable issue is what my father told me a few days before he died. He said "my lying here in this bed of affliction is a mistake. I knew that I had a problem years ago and I did nothing about it." The prostate cancer eventually spread from his prostate, to his bones, to his spine, and to his head. My father got a chance to see all of his grandchildren but he did not see them graduate from junior high school. I don't know how many more years my dad would have lived had he gotten his prostate examined and treated, but it sure would have been nice to have him around longer.

I don't want your children or your

grandchildren to miss out on their legacy and lessons with you. Nor do I wish for them to lose you prematurely.

You may or may not have great financial means for your children. If you do, terrific. But what good is money if you are not around to experience the things with your children that it can buy? That is why it is so important to have your prostate examined. If you don't have a great deal of money, there is something you can do that has more value. You can be a dream guardian for your children. Allowing your children to dream and pursue their dreams will make them goal oriented and give them purpose. Your job as a dream guardian is to expose your children to science fairs, take them to museums, take them to plays, take them to sporting events, introduce them to reading and discussions of books, and introduce them to activities where the possibilities are endless. How can you effectively do this if you leave here prematurely? Prostate cancer is treatable if detected early.

MY DEFINING MOMENT

Getting my prostate examined symbolically led to a defining moment in my life. The initial exam itself took less than five seconds but the results were life changing. What I mean by a defining moment is an activity or experience that took me to a new upper level in life. A defining moment made me view life different than previously. It changed my perspective. This defining moment made me appreciate the journey of the trials which lead up to that moment. I no longer take life for granted. At a moment's notice, the status of life could change. Longevity of life is no longer promised to the young or middle age.

My defining moment was finding out I had cancer, and by the grace of God, beating it. I remember awaiting the uncertainty of my biopsy report. Once the results came back positive, I remember awaiting the anxiety of my bone scan report to see if the cancer had begun to spread. I did not ask God "why me" because I had friends who did not live to see 40 years old due to illnesses. The bible says it rains on the just and the unjust so when I received the diagnosis, I assumed it was my time to open my umbrella. But I did ask God what I was to learn from this ordeal. The answer that I felt in my heart was to look around at other men in similar situations and inspire and encourage them. If men are uncomfortable talking about this health issue in a large forum, then I suggest they discuss it is small cell groups, or on a one-on-one basis. Fear and ignorance exists in silence. Help and the opportunity of the truth exist in open communication.

How did I handle the possibility of side effects? It is a day by day, step by step faith walk and because I know the Lord, I decided to act like it. I am scarred but not broken. I was refined by the fire but not incinerated. This challenge was an opportunity to grow as a person. God's goodness over my life prevented me from becoming depressed. I have a mindset. I choose to believe in divine healing. The same way you can go to bed feeling well and wake up feeling awful only to get news from a doctor that you have an inoperable tumor is the same way, just that quick, God can turn things around. I try to flow in God's sovereignty and trust that He knows how to navigate the ship. I'm just His passenger enjoying the ride. I am not the host of the party, I am just an invited guest. There are times when there is smooth sailing and I can walk about. There are other times when the waters are rough and I have to buckle up and let him control the journey. Life is a wonderful journey. Enjoy the ride and learn something from all your experiences. Go in good health.

**PROSTATE CANCER IS TREATABLE
IF DETECTED EARLY.**

TO CONTACT DURAND:

Durand is available for speaking engagements at events regarding his experience with prostate cancer. To reach Durand through e-mail, contact **YarrahPropertiesInc@gmail.com**

Also, like us on **Facebook** at **YarrahProp**

www.ingramcontent.com/pod-product-compliance
Lightning Source LLC
Chambersburg PA
CBHW060643280326
41933CB00012B/2134